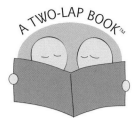

The Sunshine on My Face

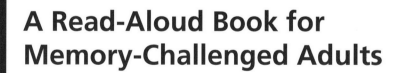

A Read-Aloud Book for Memory-Challenged Adults

by Lydia Burdick
ILLUSTRATED BY JANE FREEMAN

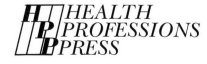

HEALTH
PROFESSIONS
PRESS

In loving memory of my parents, Shirley and Larry Burdick

"i carry your heart (i carry it in my heart)
i am never without it" —e.e.cummings

I love you for loving me the way you did.
I love you, Mom, for reading this book out loud with me.
I love you, Dad, for how beautifully you took care of Mom through her Alzheimer's.

In memory of Carolyn Handsome, our aide. Thank you for your wonderful care of Mom and Dad.

§

With all my love to my partner, Michael Bucher; my siblings and their spouses, Annie Burdick Berman and Brian Berman, Linsey Will and Bill Burdick, and Vivian Burdick and Evan Ahern; and my nieces and nephews, Julie, Evan, Josh, David, Daniel, Emily, and Alexis.

With heartfelt appreciation to—

Our home aides, Sheila Handsome, Carolyn ("Carolyn Two") Davidson, Lizette Cartegena, and Alicia Thierrens.

The Alzheimer's Caregivers' Support Group at the New York University School of Medicine's Silberstein Institute for Aging and Dementia, led by senior family counselors Emma Shulman and Gert Steinberg. Dad loved your program.

The Cabrini Hospice staff of Cabrini Medical Center in Manhattan, especially our nurses, Barbara Anderson, Greg Estrella, Maureen Madden, Eddie Rivera, and Carol Rubino, and our social worker, Ann Palmer.

—Lydia Burdick

———————

To my aunts, Ethel Cassel and Carol Cassel, with my love.

—Jane Freeman

From the Author

There is something intimate and magical about reading a book together. You can have this pleasure with a loved one with memory loss by using this read-aloud book. The words and pictures relate to most people's lives, present and past.

I wrote this book for my mother, who was diagnosed with Alzheimer's disease, to read out loud with me. I wanted to give her words to say and for us to have a happy activity to do together.

Initially, I didn't know if my mother would read these sentences either to herself, out loud to me, or at all. It was an experiment, and the experiment worked! I sat next to my mother, the book covering our two laps. I prompted my mother to read each sentence out loud. My mother, who had not spoken more than monosyllables for the last 3 years of her life, did read the sentences out loud to me. She also answered the questions I asked her about the words and illustrations.

After my mother read to me, "I love to take a warm bath and get squeaky clean," she looked intently at the accompanying drawing. When I asked her what her favorite part of the picture was, she pointed to the woman in the bathtub. "What is she doing?" I asked. My mother, a woman who loved taking baths, said "Soaking." "Oh," I said. "Who else likes to soak?" She looked at me and said "I do!" and gave me a smile that made my day.

May you find similar rewards in sharing this book.

—Lydia Burdick

How to Use This Book

GETTING STARTED

Tell your senior that you have a book that you think he or she would enjoy, and sit down together.

READING

When possible, invite your senior to read the words to you. You might say: "Mom, I'd love you to read this page to me" or "Mr. Smith, I'll read this page and you read the next, okay?" If you don't initially get a response, be patient. Ask him or her more than once to read the page.

Another way to use this book is to read the words out loud together. Or if your senior does not wish to read, or is not able to read, then read the book out loud to him or her.

You will probably find yourself using this book again and again; to keep your interactions fresh, conversation prompts are provided on pages 20–21. You may only have time or interest to read a few pages—even reading just one is fine.

LOOKING AT THE ILLUSTRATIONS

Take time to enjoy the pictures and talk about what you both see.

TALKING ABOUT THE WORDS AND PICTURES

Talk with your senior about the sentences and drawings. Ask questions about both.

ADDITIONAL IDEAS

This book can also be shared long distance by phone. It can be a thrill to hear the voice of a loved one in this manner.

Happy reading—have an enjoyable and meaningful time together!

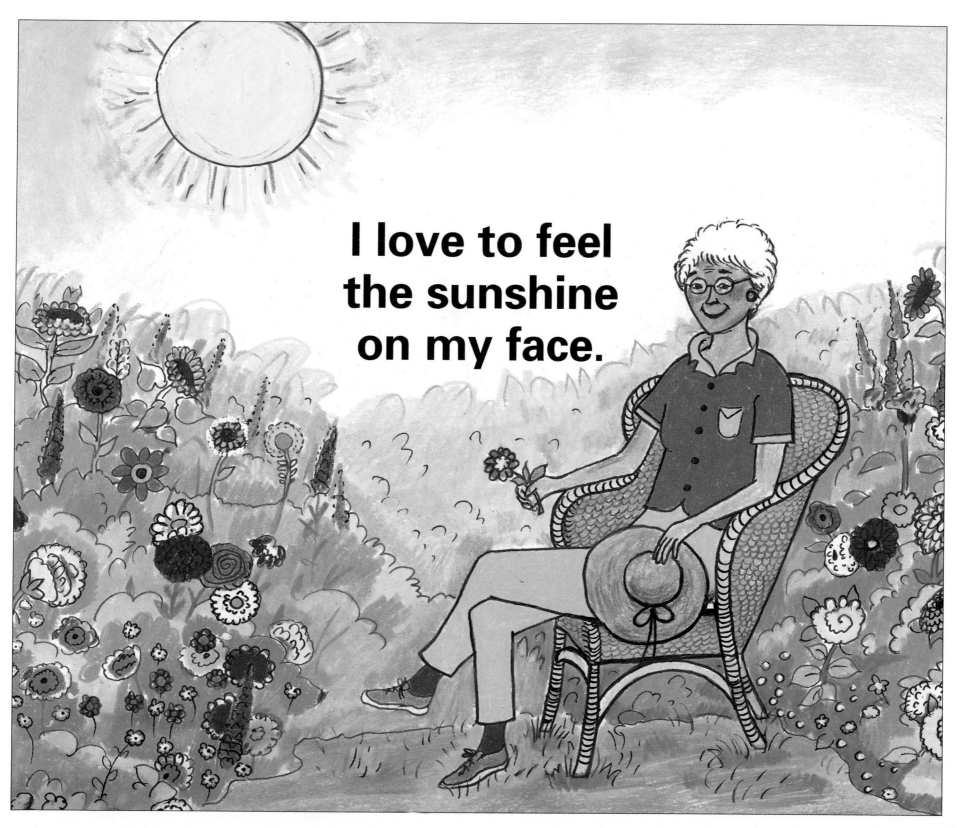

I love to feel
the sunshine
on my face.

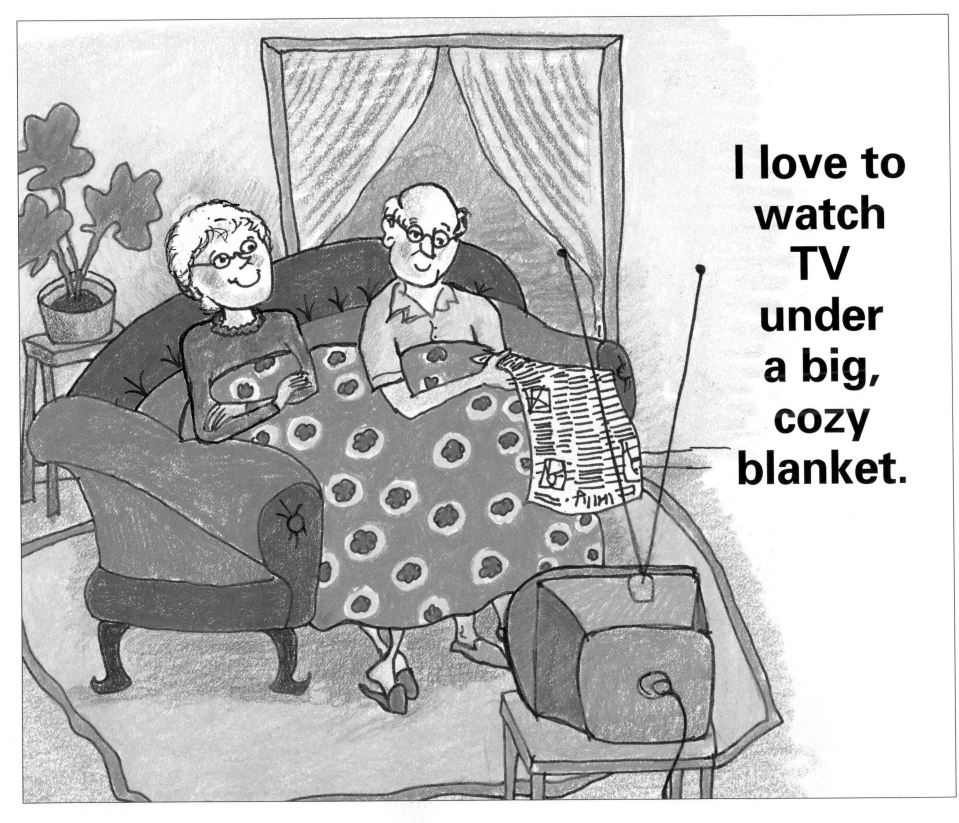

I love to watch TV under a big, cozy blanket.

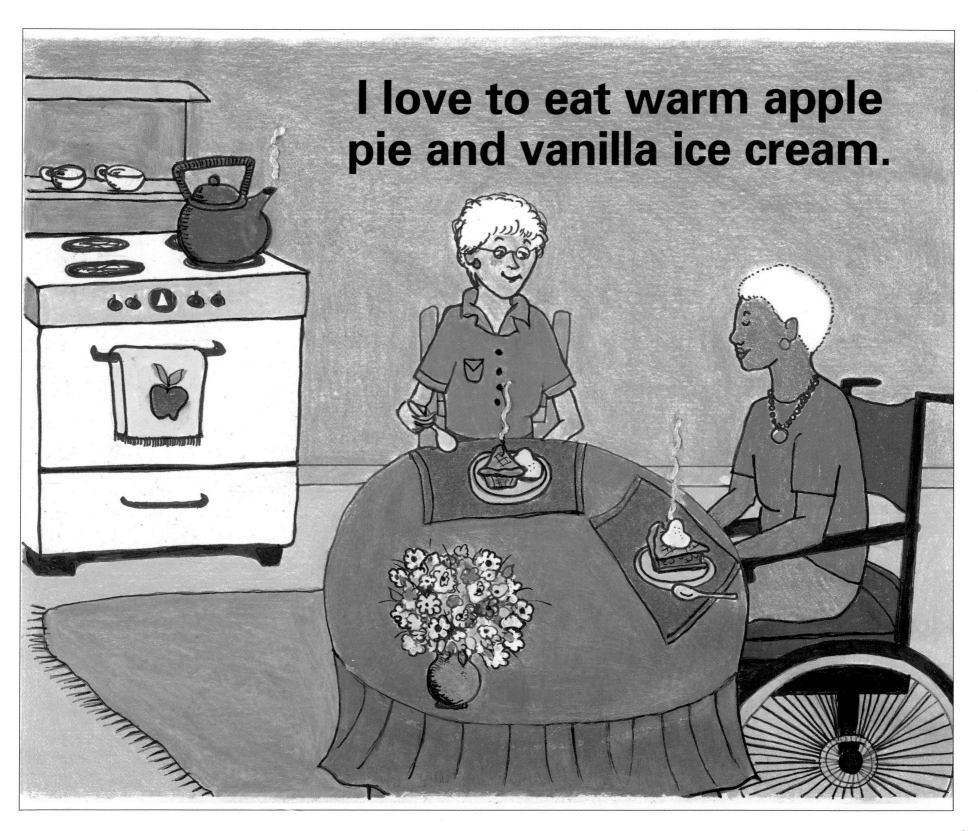

I love to eat warm apple pie and vanilla ice cream.

I love to go for a drive

in the countryside.

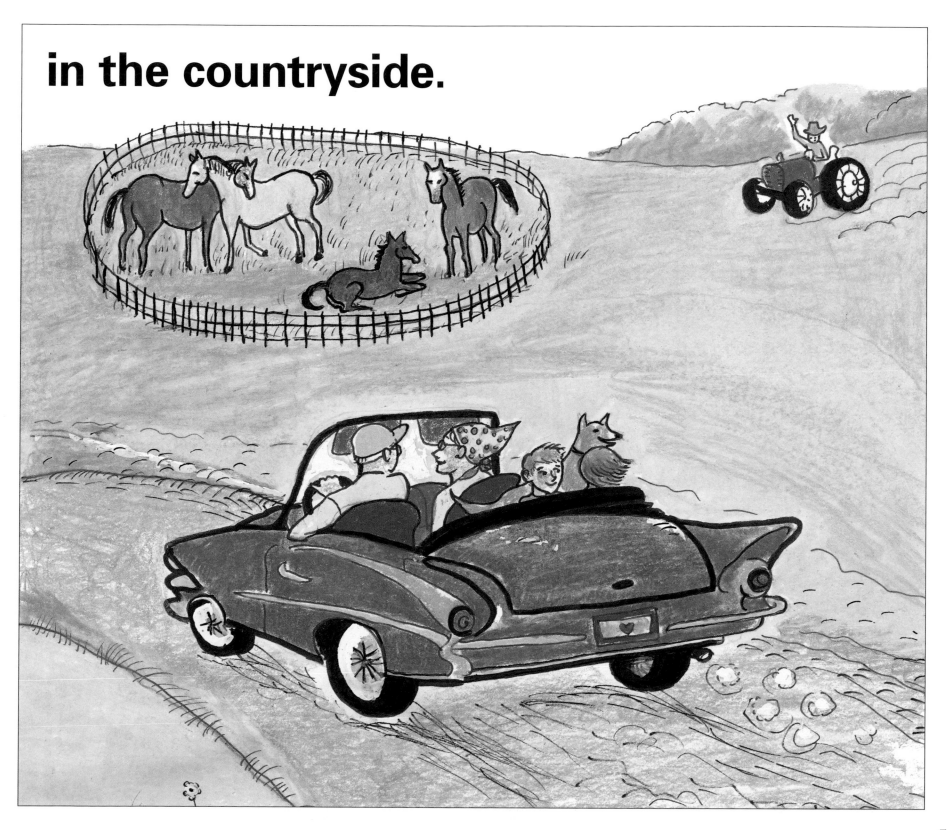

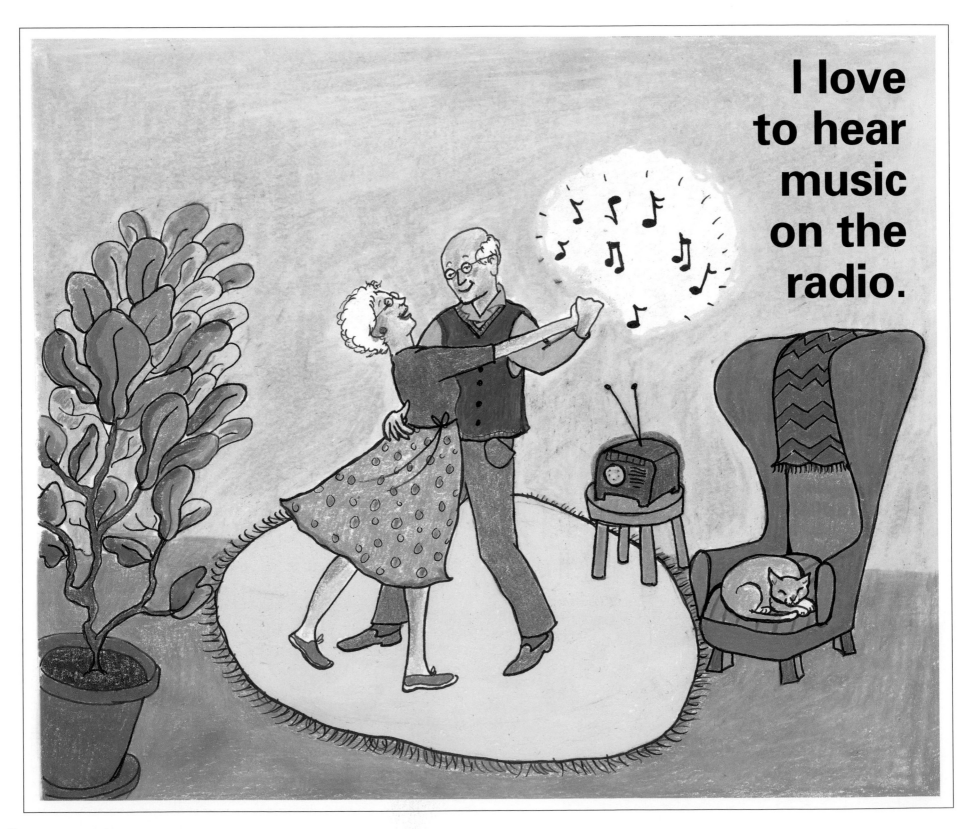

I love to hear music on the radio.

I love
to take
a warm
bath
and get
squeaky
clean.

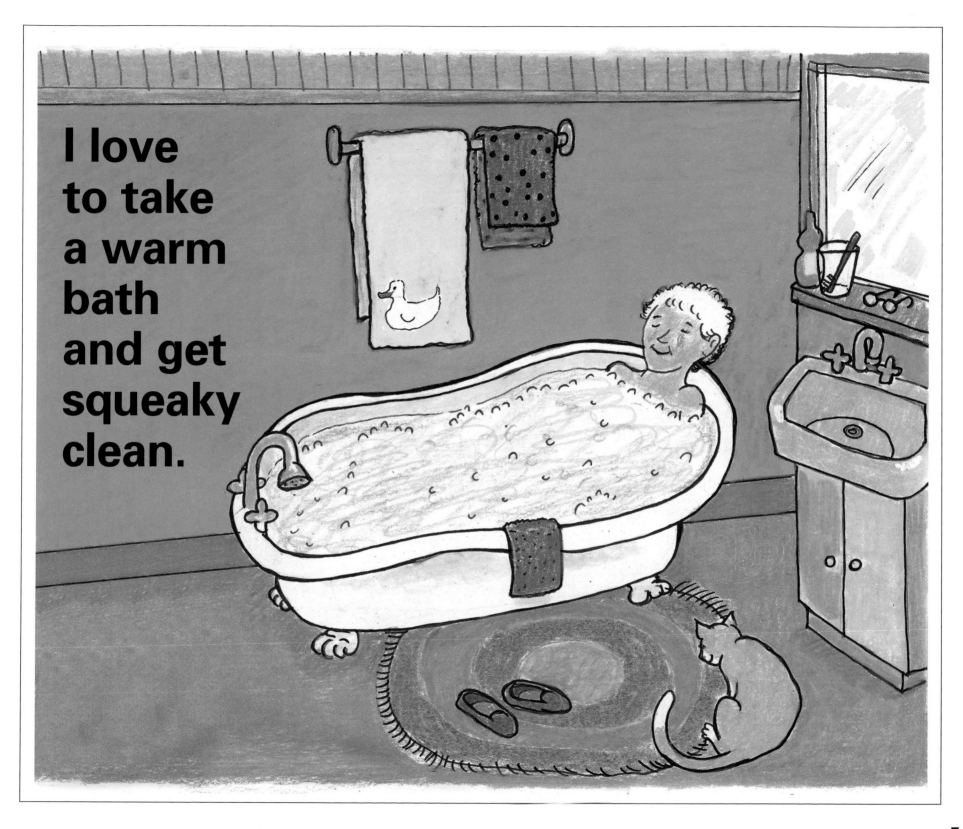

I love
to take
a nap
in the
afternoon.

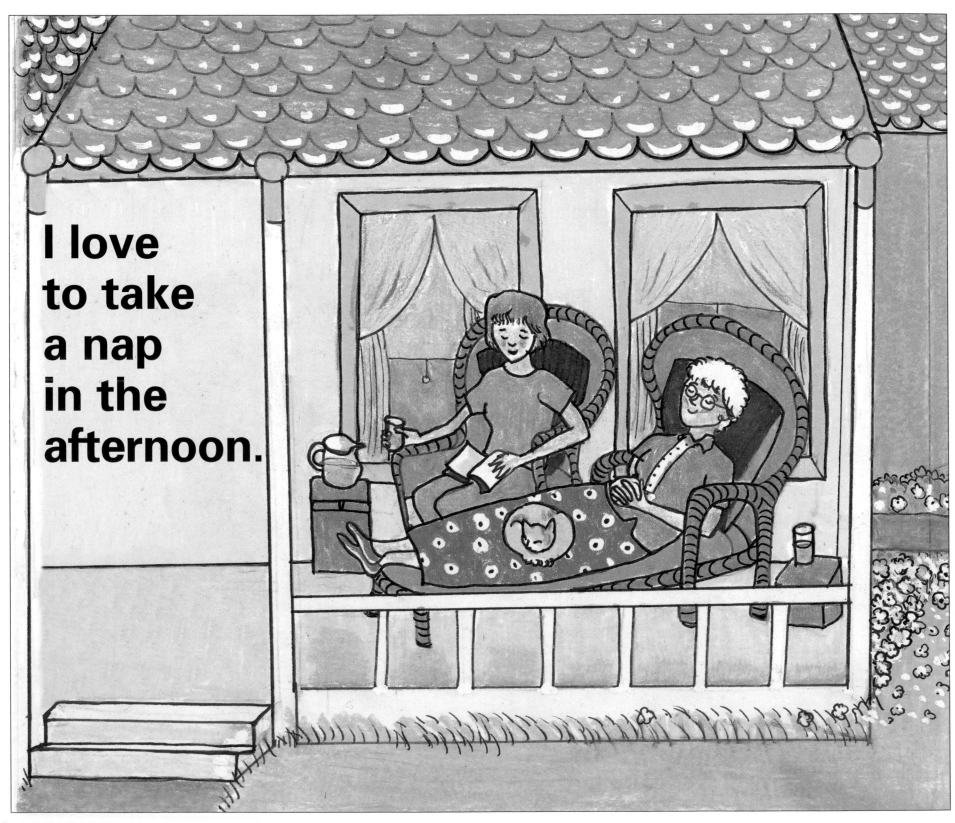

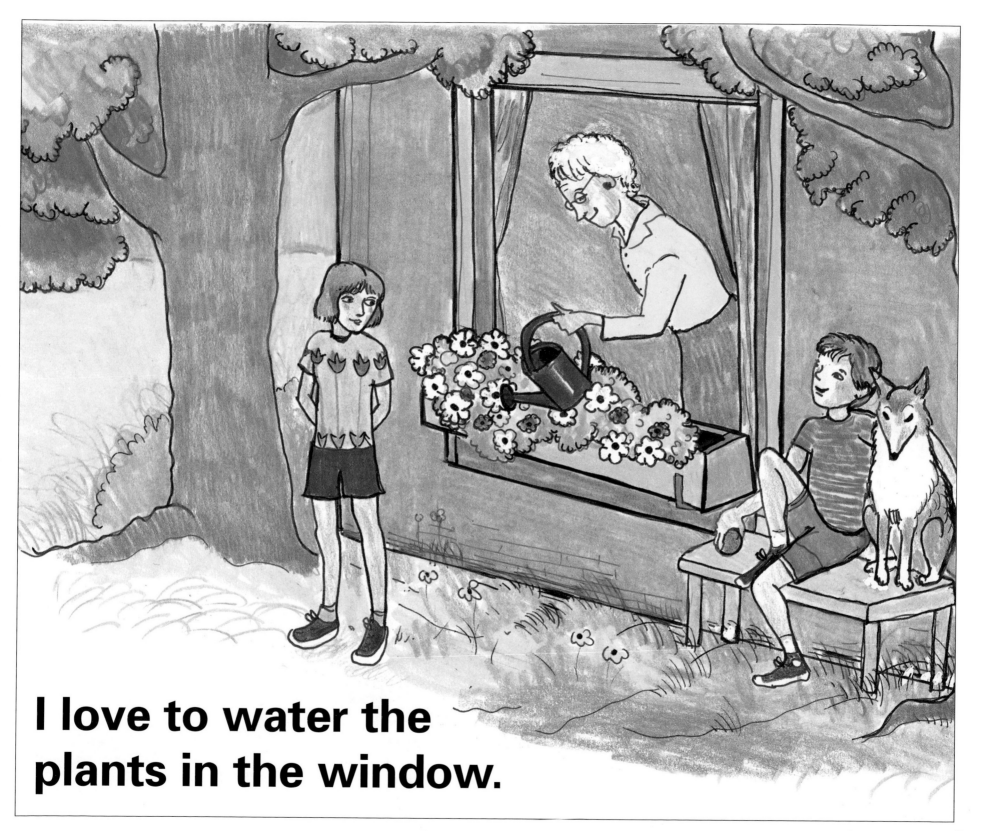

I love to water the
plants in the window.

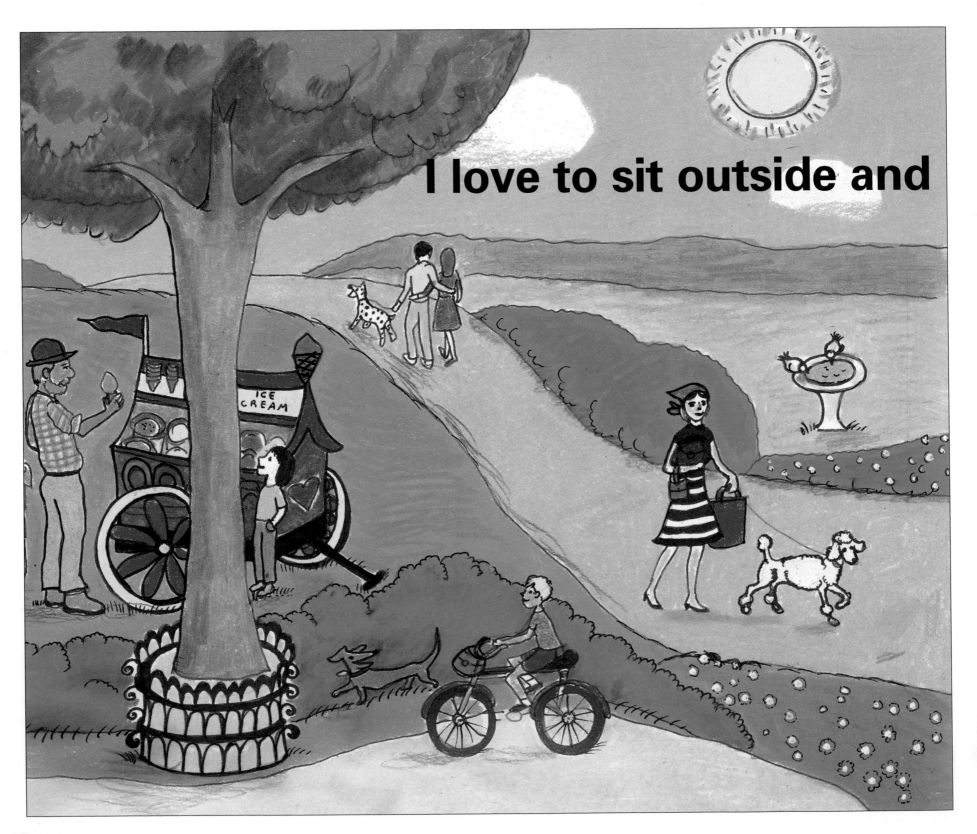

I love to sit outside and

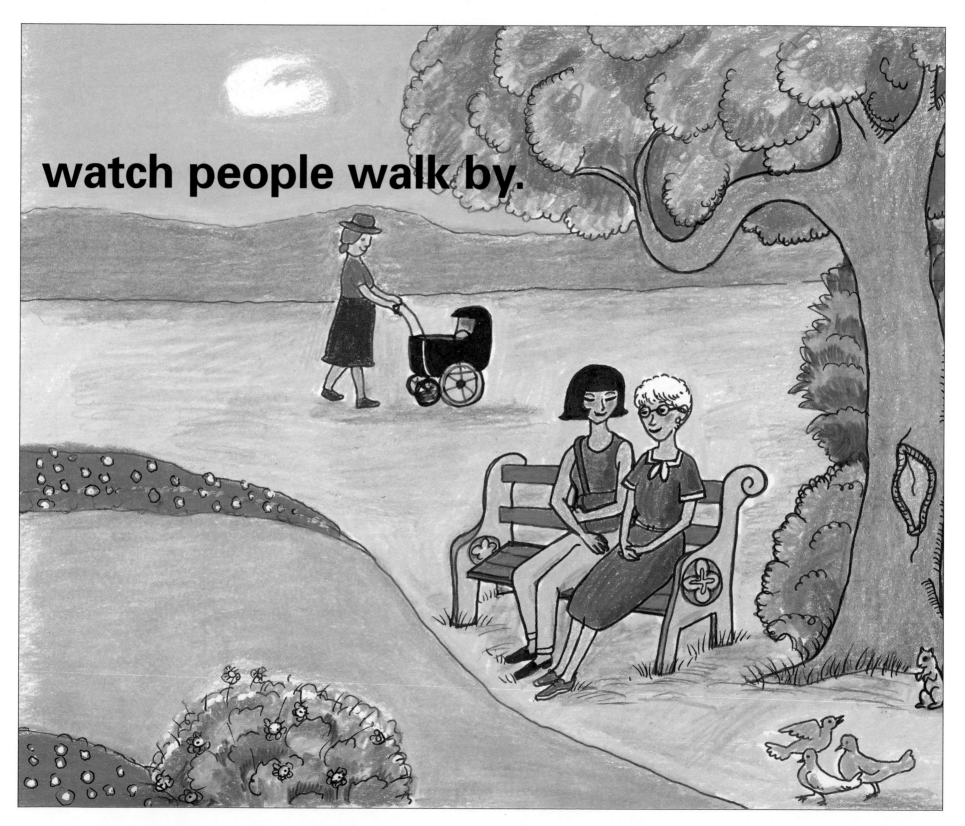

watch people walk by.

I love to sing "Happy Birthday to You."

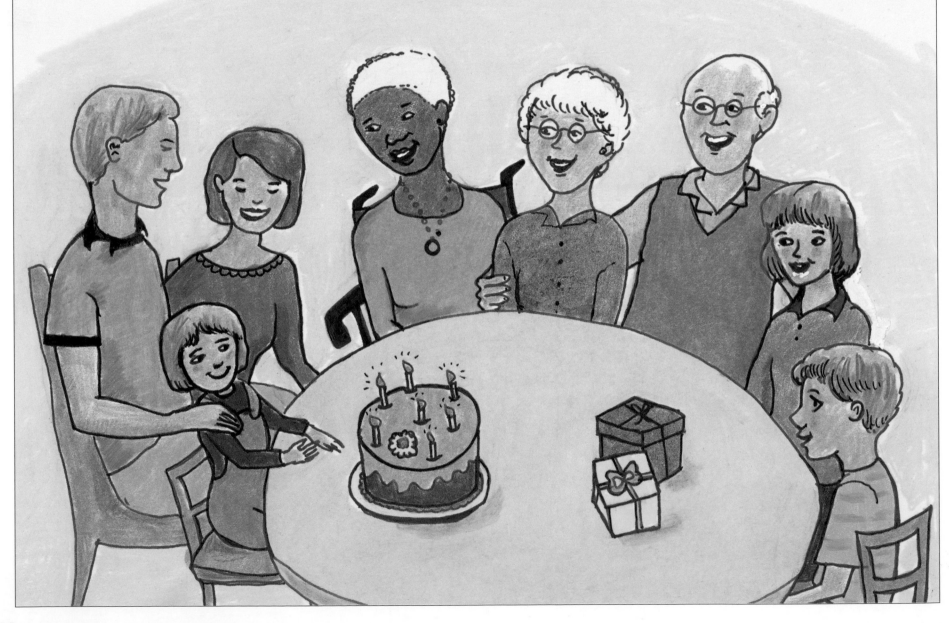

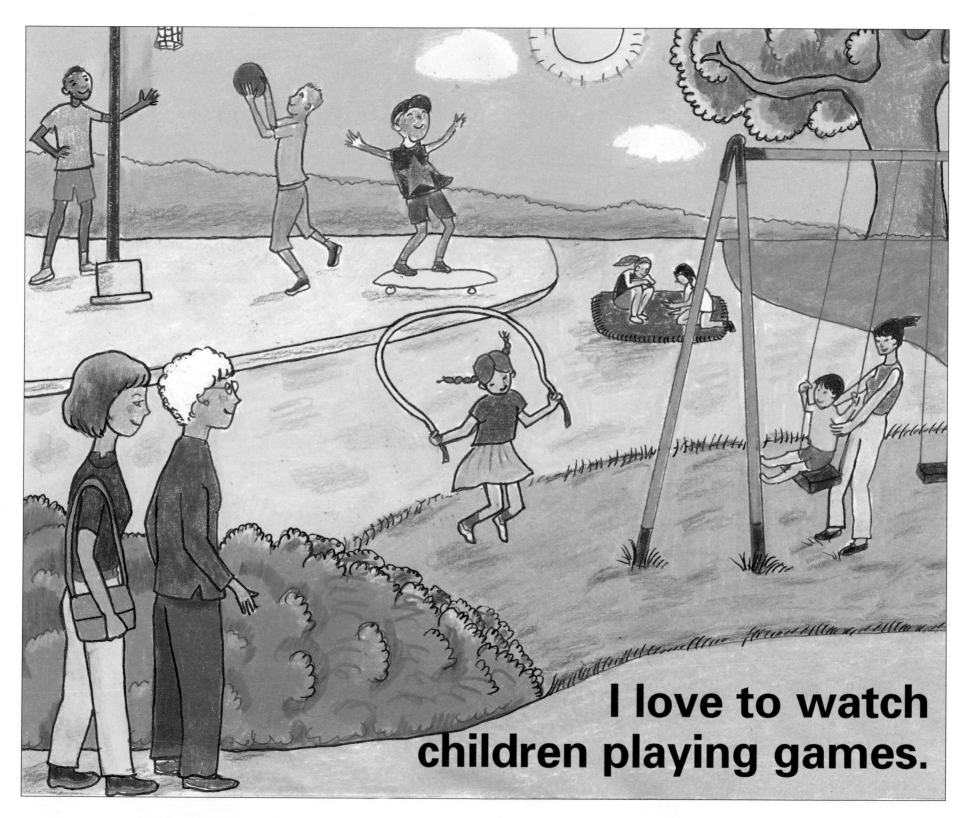

I love to watch children playing games.

I love to talk with my family

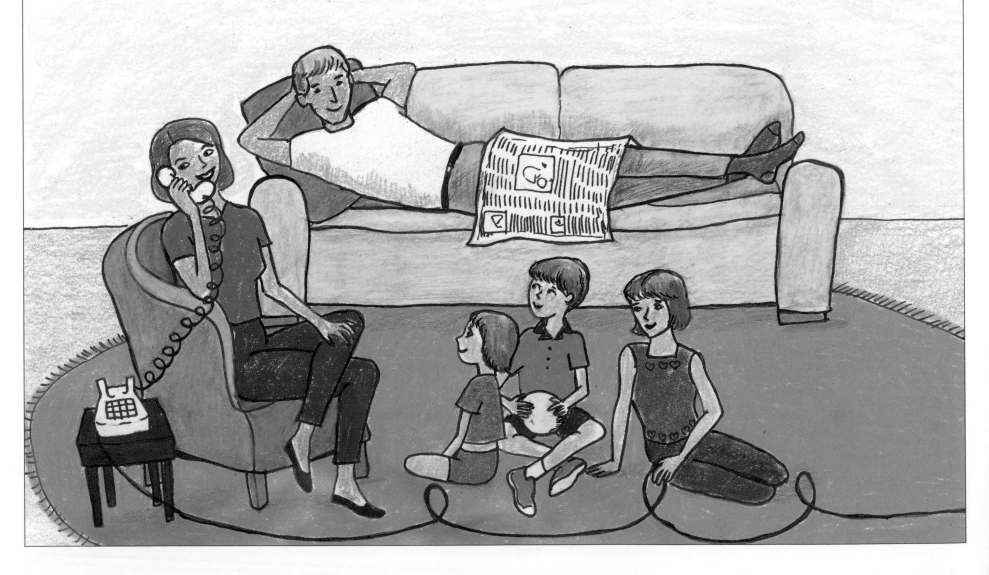

on the telephone.

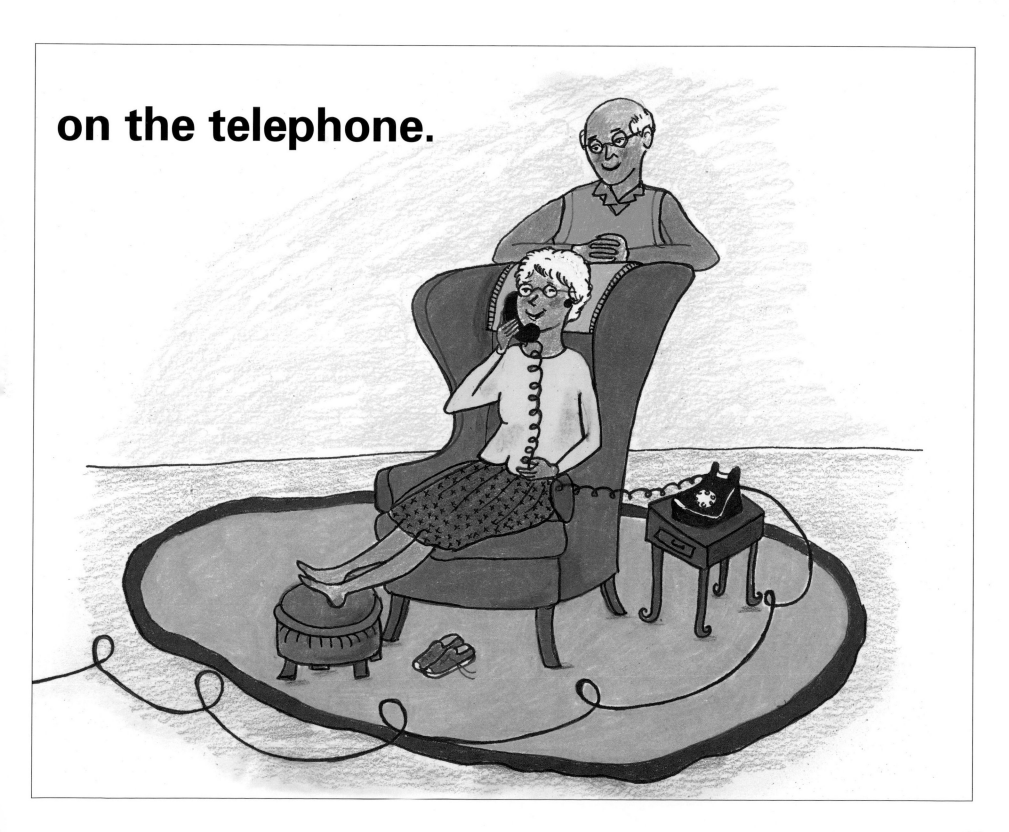

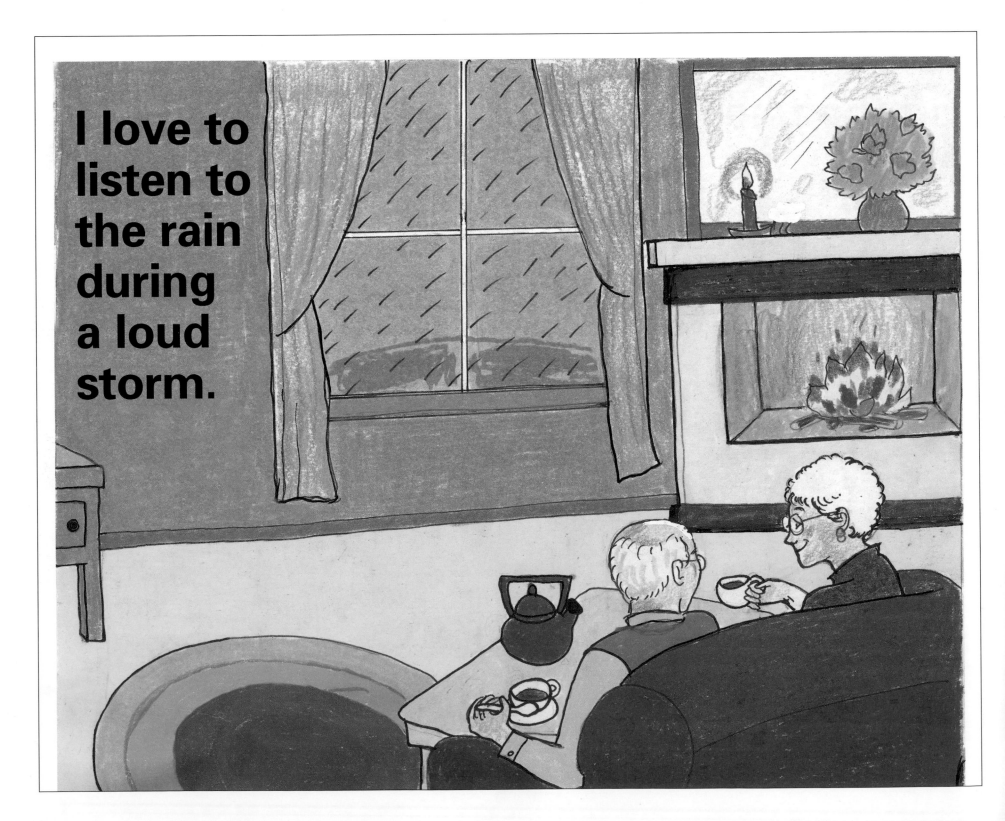

I love to
listen to
the rain
during
a loud
storm.

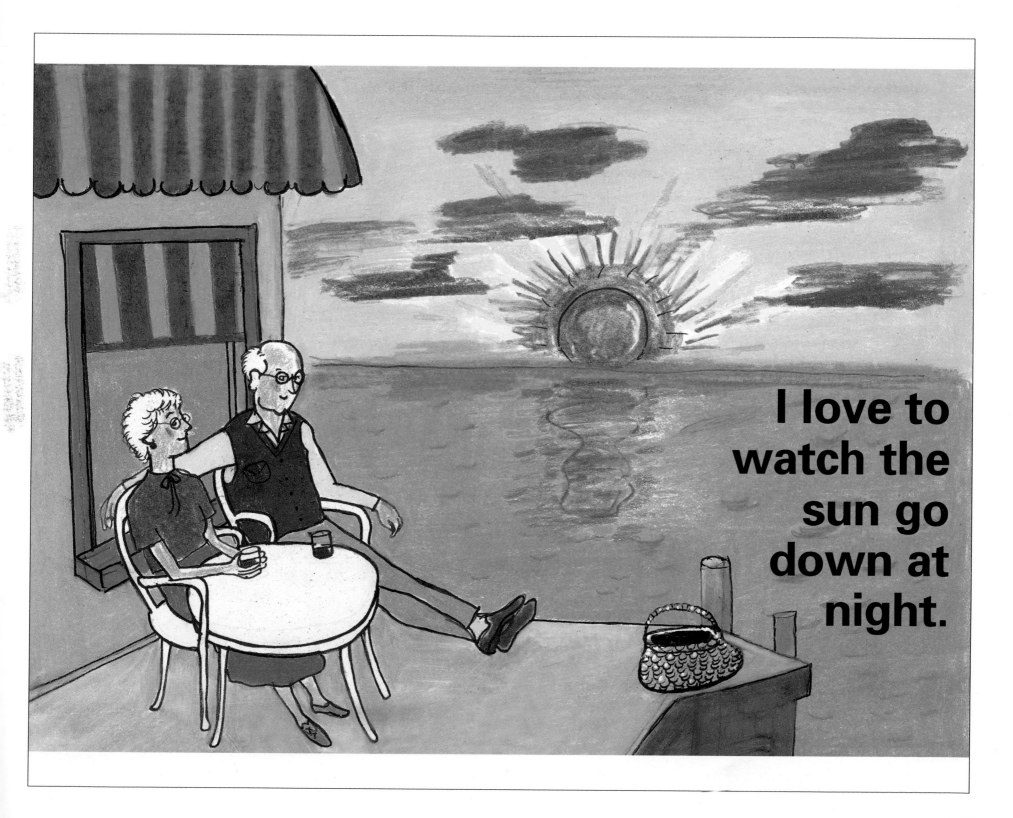

I love to watch the sun go down at night.

I love to
be hugged
by someone
I love.

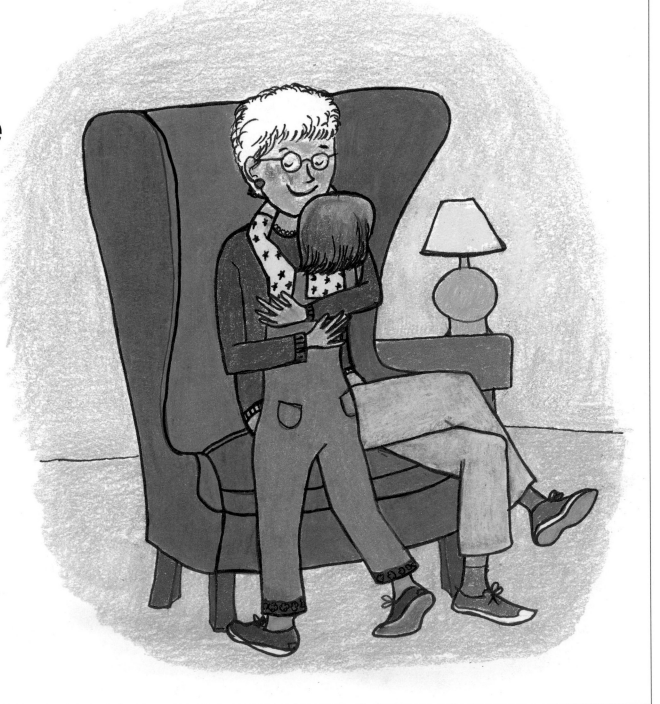

I love to read this book out loud with you!

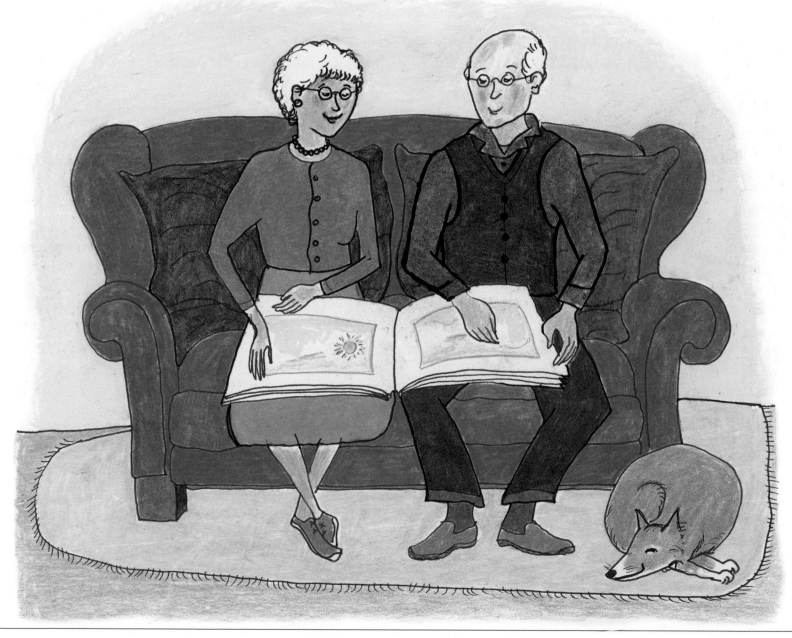

CONVERSATION PROMPTS—prompts useful for all pages

Questions about the illustrations:

> What do you like in the drawing?
> What are the different objects you see?
> What are the people or animals doing?
> Do you like to do what the people in the pictures are doing?

Questions about the sentences:

> Do you love/like to do the activity?
> Have you done the activity in the past?
> Would you like to do it in the future?
> Would you like to do it now/later? *(Ask only if the activity is a viable option.)*

CONVERSATION PROMPTS—prompts useful for specific pages

page 1   I love to feel the sunshine on my face.

> Do you love/like to feel the sunshine on your face?
> How does the sun feel on your face?
> Where do you feel the sunshine? *(gently touch face)*
> What do you like to do outside?

page 2   I love to watch TV under a big, cozy blanket.

> Do you love/like to watch TV?
> Do you have a big, cozy blanket? What does it look like?
> What TV shows have you enjoyed?
> Do you remember when your family got a television set?

page 3   I love to eat warm apple pie and vanilla ice cream.

> Do you love/like to eat apple pie? Vanilla ice cream?
> Do you like the smell of apple pie?
> What is your favorite dessert (or pie)?
> What is your favorite flavor of ice cream?
> What else do you like to eat?

pages 4–5   I love to go for a drive in the countryside.

> Do you love/like to go for a drive in the countryside?
> What do you see when you go for a drive in the countryside?
> What else do you see?
> Where do you like to go in the car?
> Who do you like to visit when you go for a drive?
> What kind of car have you had? What color was it?

page 6   I love to hear music on the radio.

> Do you love/like to listen to music?
> What kind of music do you like?
> Did you ever play a musical instrument?
> Do you like to dance when you hear music?
> Would you like to dance now?

page 7   I love to take a warm bath and get squeaky clean.

> Do you love/like to take a bath?
> Do you prefer taking a shower?
> Do you like bathing in the morning or at night?
> What is your favorite part of bathing? Your least favorite part?

page 8   I love to take a nap in the afternoon.

> Do you love/like to take naps?
> Where do you like to take your nap?
> How do you feel when you get up after a nap?

page 9   I love to water the plants in the window.

> Do you love/like to water the plants?
> What are your favorite plants/flowers?
> Did you ever have a garden?
> What did you grow in your garden?

pages 10–11   I love to sit outside and watch people walk by.

Do you love/like to sit outside? Where?
Who do you see when you sit outside?
What do people do when they are outside?
Would you like to take a walk later?

page 12   I love to sing "Happy Birthday to You."

Do you love/like to celebrate birthdays?
What kind of food do you eat at a birthday party?
What is the best part of having a birthday?
Do you like to sing?
Would you like to sing "Happy Birthday" with me now?
What is your favorite song? Would you sing it with me now?

page 13   I love to watch children playing games.

Do you love/like to watch children playing games?
Is there a special child in your life?
Do you have children of your own?
What games did you like to play when you were a child?

pages 14–15   I love to talk with my family on the telephone.

Do you love/like to talk on the telephone with your family and
friends?
Who do you like to talk to on the phone?
Would you like to call someone on the phone now?

page 16   I love to listen to the rain during a loud storm.

Do you like to listen to the rain?
Do you like storms?
Do you like to be outside when it's raining?
What do you wear when you go out in the rain?

page 17   I love to watch the sun go down at night.

Do you love/like to watch the sun go down at night?
What color is the sky when the sun sets?
What is your favorite thing about sunsets?
What evening activities do you do to get ready for bed?

page 18   I love to be hugged by someone I love.

Do you love being hugged?
Who would you love to be hugged by right now?
Who else do you love to hug?
How does it feel to be hugged?

page 19   I love to read this book out loud with you!

Who do you love to read this book out loud with?
Do you love to read this book out loud with me?
Do you love to read books?
What is your favorite book?
Would you like to read this book again? Now? Later? Tomorrow?
Who would you like to read this book with next time?

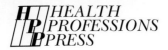

Health Professions Press
Post Office Box 10624
Baltimore, MD 21285-0624
U.S.A.

www.healthpropress.com

A Two-Lap Book™ is a trademark owned by Lydia Burdick.

Library of Congress catalog number: RC523.2.B874 2004.
616.8'31'00222—dc22
ISBN 1-932529-09-8

Printed in Hong Kong.

Illustrated by Jane Freeman.

Two-Lap Books™ are available at a quantity discount with bulk purchases for educational, therapeutic, and human services programs. For information, please write to: SPECIAL SALES DEPARTMENT, HEALTH PROFESSIONS PRESS, POST OFFICE BOX 10624, BALTIMORE, MD 21285 or fax 410-337-8539.

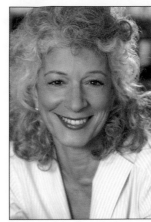

Photograph by Steve Ladner.

With a master's degree in Clinical Practices (psychology), **Lydia Burdick's** career has been in human resources. Since 1993, she has been a consultant at an international outplacement firm. Lydia wrote *The Sunshine on My Face* in the course of caring for her mother who was diagnosed with Alzheimer's disease. "One of my greatest pleasures," she says, "was sitting next to my mother and hearing her read the words from this book when she had stopped speaking almost completely."